YOU DON'T HAVE TO BE TO BE RICH & FAMOUS TO LOSE WEIGHT!

YOU DON'T HAVE TO BE RICH & FAMOUS TO LOSE WEIGHT!

Beverly L. Jackson

To order additional copies of this book, contact:
Xlibris Corporation
1-888-795-4274
www.Xlibris.com
Orders@Xlibris.com
69594

TABLE OF CONTENTS

FOREWORD

For those of you who picked up this book hoping to find a quick fix to your weight loss problems, I want you to know right now: THIS IS NOT THE BOOK FOR YOU !!!

This book DOES NOT show you how to lose the pounds and inches in a couple weeks. This book DOES NOT show you how to drop the weight without moving a muscle. And most important, this book DOES NOT GIVE YOU FALSE HOPE !!!

What this book does do is give you practical, everyday, sound advice on how to lose the weight and keep it off for the rest of your life. This book will speak to your specific needs and what YOU need to do to be successful. This book will teach you that nothing comes without a price and if it does, it's not worth the effort.

Losing weight and maintaining weight loss is a process. It's a process that takes time AND effort. It takes hard work and a commitment to yourself and to your future. It takes discipline and dedication. But with hard work and dedication come accomplishment and life changing results.

How bad do you want it? How hard are you willing to work? If this is you, then THIS IS DEFINITELY THE BOOK FOR YOU!! Let's get started. The rest of your life is waiting and you don't have time to waste.

Beverly L. Jackson
Author

ATTENTION GENTLEMEN

Just in case you picked up this book and were trying to decide if this was a book you might want to read, I'm here to tell you that it definitely is. While the verbiage of my book is pretty much geared to women—simply because I am a woman and that's what I know the most about—I don't want that to be the reason you choose NOT to read it. I believe that everything I talk about in these pages is just as important for men as it is for women. We are all different. We are all individuals. And we all must find what works best for us when it comes to weight loss and weight management.

If you buy my book, start to read it and find that it really isn't for you, let me suggest that you pass it on to a female friend. I'm sure she will not only find the book valuable for her, but she'll probably think you're a pretty neat guy for giving it to her!

Whatever you decide, I hope you will purchase my book and give it a read. It's not filled with frilly, girly, sissy stuff, if that's what you're worried about. I've tried to make it down-to-earth, straight forward, and honest, no matter who reads it.

CHAPTER 1

Setting the Ground Rules

I'm really tired of seeing all of those books out there, written by famous actors and actresses that talk about how they lost weight. Like they've got some special secret that only they found out about and now you have to read their book if you want to do the same. Well, I'm here to tell you that there's no special secret. They don't have the market cornered on how to lose weight. In fact, most of them have lost those same pounds over and over and over and over again. Only this time, they decided that even if it doesn't work permanently—because none of the other times did either—they're at least going to make some money telling you about it. And the part that bothers me the most is that we, the unrich and unfamous public, believe that just because they did it with this one particular diet, we should be able to do it too . . . as if their current success is a guarantee of ours. Ladies, come on. We're better then that.

I don't want to take away from them the hard work they may have put into their current success. But, you and I both know they are famous and have a lot of money, so when they decide to do something like lose weight, they just go ahead and do it. And the media is always there to record their amazing efforts and give them all the credit for doing it. They buy the most expensive workout clothes because they have to look good. They buy the best equipment or pay for the best trainer because—well, because they can afford it. None of that takes any thought or effort or commitment on their part, at least, not to get started. And if they get off track or lose momentum, well, they've got this trainer that will keep them on track, at least until the desired weight is lost.

And why exactly are they losing the weight anyway? They probably need the publicity or need to make themselves more available for better roles. They've gotten older or out of shape and they just don't look as good as they use to and so, they're not as marketable as they use to be. They're not going to stay famous and rich for very long if they are no longer marketable, are they? They have motives that would get most of us started I think.

It's not my desire to bash famous people that have lost weight. The point I am trying to make is that they are human beings just like you and me. They have some options available to them that most of us don't have, but that doesn't mean we can't be just as successful—or even MORE successful.

So, let's get back to what's important here—You and I. We are everyday people. We are not rich. We are not famous. We are not trying to jumpstart our career or even get our pictures on the front cover of some well-known magazine. We are just people who get up and go to work for a living and make just enough money to pay the bills and have a little bit of fun once in awhile. We are basically happy people, but over the years we've managed to put on a few extra pounds or gotten off track of staying fit and in shape and the older years are creeping up on us. We don't look quite like we use to, we don't feel like we use to and we can't seem to eat like we use to. We can't "pig out" whenever we want and expect nothing to happen. We find ourselves being a little more careful with what we do eat because our bodies are not responding to the nourishment we take in like before.

This book is not just for women. If you're a man and you've decided to give this a try, wonderful! I'm behind you 100%, but I want to be very honest and upfront with you right from the start. I don't know a thing about a man's body and how it works. I'm a woman and the things I'm writing about are because I've done them, I've tried them, I am living proof that they work—for women! I would suspect that just about everything I talk about on these pages will work for anyone, man or woman, and any age, young and old. I don't want the fact that this book is geared to women to keep you from reading what I have to say. I believe you will get valuable information that will help you to be successful in your weight loss and weight management efforts. Man and woman!

Women's bodies have unique principles that just seem to take over our lives as we get older. I'm here to tell you that all the things my older friends use to tell me about "once you turn 40" are absolutely true. I believed them back then, but it was one of those things that I figured I'd deal with when the time came.

Well, sister—the time is NOW! You have to want to be successful. You have to want to set new goals and change your life permanently and for the better. It is always so easy to put off today what you can do tomorrow, but I have learned that we are never guaranteed tomorrow. It is what you do with your life today that will make the difference. Don't keep putting off those things you want for yourself. As you get older, time seems to go so much faster and before you know it, it's all behind you and there are no more tomorrows. Let's make a difference today and if we do, those tomorrows will be even better!

THE FIRST AND MOST IMPORTANT STEP TOWARD SUCCESS IS THE FEELING THAT WE CAN SUCCEED.

Nelson Boswell

CHAPTER 2

How to Get Started

Listen to me ladies! After 40, a woman's body starts to do things you never thought possible. If you had a waist before 40, you can be sure that you won't have one after 40! And for those of you reading my book who are still young and in complete denial, take the following words to heart: Work hard at keeping your abs as tight as possible while you're young because after 40, trust me, you will work twice as hard and see half the results—if that! And I'm not talking about just those women who get pregnant and have a family. This applies to ALL women, no matter what we do or don't do with our bodies.

For women, everything begins to settle around the midsection, if it hasn't already started before you hit 40. Your metabolism slows down so the same amount of exercise and activity reaps half the affect as before. Not to mention the aches and pains. I remember the moment I turned 40, I hurt from the top of my head to the bottom of my feet, and it lasted for a full 9 years until I turned 50!! I'm serious. Every day was a chore just to get up and get moving. The thought of anything except normal walking to and from somewhere was simply out of the question. But, believe me when I tell you that no matter how much you hurt or how hard it may be to exercise, it is so very important to make the effort. And you have to start now!

Throughout this book, the basic theme will be E-X-E-R-C-I-S-E. Everything else I share with you is important, but without exercise, you may as well not even start. I have learned that the exercise piece is what makes everything else easier and worthwhile. If you can put 30 minutes of some form of exercise into your day to day routine, you are on your way to a healthier and much happier you.

I remember when I started my program. My mind and my body were so totally in sync, I knew that there was absolutely nothing out there that would affect how I was feeling and what I was doing. I was strong. I was in charge. I was confident . . . . I was in for a very big surprise. The company that I work for is big on junk food. It seems like daily you can walk into the break room and there will be something on the table that just calls out to you. One day there were Krispy Krème Donuts. The next day there were cookies, M&M's (my personal favorites), cake, pie, you name it, it was sitting there just waiting for me. Almost calling to me. I needed every ounce of strength I had to resist the temptation and you know what? I did! And every time I went into that break room and saw that "stuff" on the table, I simply turned around and walked out. Eventually, I was able to resist with little or no effort. You see, the accomplishments that came out of my perseverance were so much more rewarding than a fleeting indulgence of something sweet. I have a sweet tooth that just won't quit, so giving that up on a regular basis has been extremely hard for me. But I have found some wonderful substitutes that satisfy me just as much and even more since I know they're better for me. I'll share some of my tasty finds a little later in the book. Right now we need to set the groundwork and get you started on *your very last weight loss program.*

Okay. Let me break this down for you. I'm going to tell you what I did, how I did it, and then I'm going to share my results with you. Nowhere in these pages will I tell you that any of this is easy. It's not, so get that out of your head right now. If it were, everybody would be doing it. And it wouldn't be worth it. But it is worth it when you see the results that come from it. I thought that because I was over 50, 7 years over 50 to be exact, I thought I was never going to see the kind of results I've seen in my body, but I was wrong. I now know that it doesn't matter how old you are, how overweight you are, how out of shape you are, or even what your shape is, you can change it for the better.

The other important piece to this is that this is not dieting. Please remember that. I do not believe in dieting. The reason is that when you stop dieting, you will gain all of it back—and then some. What we are going to do here is *change behavior*. We are going to develop new habits that become a regular part of your daily life. That means that no matter what you do, it will be easier because it is a part of your daily routine. In fact, I have found that since I have been doing these things on a regular basis, I feel like something is wrong if I don't do them each and every day. My body knows what to expect from me now so it reacts either favorably or unfavorably when I do the right things and when I do the wrong things. It's almost like my physical alarm clock, if you will, that goes off if I've forgotten to eat enough or I eat too much or I haven't had enough water or I didn't exercise today. It's amazing how in tune you truly can be with your own body. And, at that point, you are the master of your destiny. From then on, the sky is the limit!

* *

Knowing is not enough; we must apply.

Willing is not enough; we must do.

Johann Wolfgang von Goethe

* *

If there were any kind of secret in weight loss, it would be this: The number of calories IN the body must be less than the number of calories OUT of the body in order for you to lose weight.

SIMPLY PUT:

 3500 calories = 1 pound

What that means to you is you must remove at least 3500 calories from your weekly intake or increase your weekly output by 3500 calories in order to lose one pound. But wait, that's great because if you work with one pound at a time, that's the pace you want. You see, if you lose weight too fast, statistics prove that you will end up gaining it back—and then some! The key is to lose it gradually. This is a total and complete lifestyle change, not a race. This is the rest of your life so you have to make it count. Besides, this is hard work and who wants to do this again and again and again? I sure don't.

I made up my mind right from the start that once I got the weight off and changed my eating habits, this was going to be it. There would be no going back. And you know what, that's exactly what I'm doing. Everything I'm sharing with you is the way I live each and every day now. The changes I have made are now habits. Good habits. And when they become habits, it's easy to keep doing it. Right? It's not difficult if it's part of your daily routine. In fact, I notice when I don't do what I'm suppose to do. That makes me more committed to getting it right tomorrow. Do you realize what that means? That means that if I choose to splurge today, I don't beat myself up about it. I just get back on track tomorrow. That means I leave no chance for those bad habits to set in again. I get right back to where I was the day before and keep going.

So, before you can reduce your weekly consumption by 3500 calories, it might be a good idea to see exactly how many calories you are currently taking in. And the only way you are going to do that is to start writing down what you eat. Believe me, once you start this, you will be amazed just how much food you are putting into your body on a daily basis. And when you know how much is going in, and exactly what is going in, then you will be better able to determine what you can reduce or eliminate all together from your daily intake.

I remember talking to a girl who was also trying to change her eating habits. She felt that she was a pretty conscientious eater and there really wasn't too much she could eliminate from her diet, but she started writing things down anyways. After about a week or so, she realized that she was stopping every morning on her way to work for a latte at her favorite coffee shop. After finding out that one 12 ounce Café Latte has 102 calories, she decided that was something she could do without for now. Just removing that one item from her weekly intake reduced her calorie count by 510. That's huge!

I talked with another girl who remembers she had to have a Snickers candy bar every afternoon around 3:00 p.m. A 2.1 ounce Snickers bar has 280 calories. One of those five days a week removed from her diet reduced her intake by 1400 calories. Wow!

Do you get the idea? It's not hard to find something in your current diet that you can do without. There may be several things you are consuming on a regular basis that are the main reasons you are unable to lose weight. What's more important? Having a latte every morning, or a candy bar every afternoon, or taking off those extra pounds you've been carrying around for the past few years and feeling ten times better because of it. Once you've mastered this program, you can have that latte or candy bar again—just not every day. Maybe once a week. Trust me when I tell you that when you do have it, it will taste even better because it's truly a treat!

Okay, so let's talk a minute about writing down what you eat. You can use whatever works best for you. Make yourself a food journal of some sort for every day of the week. You want to start recording what you eat the first 7 days so that you can get a better idea of just how many calories you are taking in before you begin to reduce that number. This is not the time to cheat or cut corners. It's imperative that you get an accurate listing and calorie count of exactly what you are eating from the moment you get up until the time you go to bed. Once you have that information, you can then decide where the changes need to start.

Below is an example of what I'm talking about. You can create something like this or make up something that works better for you. Whatever it is, it needs to show how much you're consuming, what you're consuming and how many calories are in it. There are several good websites that will help you with tracking calories. I have listed some of them in the back of the book.

SAMPLE FOOD JOURNAL

FOOD JOURNAL			
DAY _____		DATE	___/___/___
AMOUNT	*FOOD & BEVERAGES*	*CALORIES*	*COMMENTS*
	TOTAL		

Add as many lines as you want and then a place for your total at the bottom. You might want to keep track of your physical activities this same way. It's important to try to do a minimum of 180 minutes of exercise every week. Now let's take a minute to reflect on those "famous people" and their "dieting regiments". It seems like daily we read about another diet wonder that has just been discovered that will make you lose massive amounts of weight in record time.

They have been out on the market, but no one has really promoted them until now. And it's because a certain "famous person" is now sharing this with you, because it worked for them, so it must be good. Whatever he or she "famous person" is telling you about what THEY did to lose all that weight, must be the way we have to lose it . . . . , Right? Wrong! I'm here to tell you—Don't Waste Your Time!!!! The secrets they are sharing are temporary, not permanent. You may see results drastically and quickly—which, let's face it, we all want that quick fix—but it's fleeting. That's NOT the way to do it. Not the way to take it off AND keep it off. You are going to find yourself right back where you were, or worse, if you follow their recommendations. What you need is to simply change your way of thinking about food and change your behavior. Stop trying to do what other people are doing.

Every BODY is different. What works for this person may not work for that person. Results vary, don't they? What you want is something that works for **YOU**. Something specifically designed for **YOUR** body! In order to do that, you have to understand your body and what it needs and doesn't need. You have to take charge of what you consume and don't consume. And let's face it: you have to be able to say "yes" and "no" when it comes to your own personal health and wellbeing. You are in control of the destiny of what you eat, how you eat and most importantly, what you look like. Take it from me. That is what's so liberating. I no longer have to worry about if I'm going to be in an environment where I have to test my will power to resist eating or drinking something that I shouldn't. I have mastered my own destiny in this area that it's not difficult for me to say "no" to it. I can eat what I need and want, stop eating when I know it's enough, and be totally and completely satisfied with the choices I have made. How awesome is that?

Lucky for me I had been on this program long enough when the holidays rolled around. Normally, I would have been concerned about all the "goodies" that everyone was bringing into work. And then what friends would have when I went over to visit. I could walk into the break room at work or a friend's house and simply eat what was best for me. I could either resist the "goodies" or

I could choose to have a very small taste. Just enough to enjoy it, but not enough to over do it. To be perfectly honest, I find that since I don't splurge like I use to, that when I do, I really enjoy the splurge a whole lot more. I have made eating a kind of special occasion if you will. It's a time that I set aside to eat what I want when I need to. No more mindless eating. Mindless eating means that before you know it, you have consumed an entire week's worth of calories in one sitting. Then what do you do. You figure you've already blown it, so what's the sense and you just keep going down that path until you've lost sight of the track you were on. All that hard work up to that point is gone and when you finally decide it's time to stop and get back on track, you find yourself all the way back to the beginning. How awful is that? Don't you want to stop having to start all over? Don't you want to stop blowing it time after time after time? Well, as soon as you make that mind and body decision to change, that's when you will become the master of you and at that point you can keep heading in the right direction. Little slips and little splurges are just that—little. You refocus and get right back on track and progress continues.

Perseverance allows you
to get back on track
when you hit a detour.

—Catherine Pulsifer

Okay. Let's move on . . . .

CHAPTER 3

Surround Yourself with Positive Reinforcements

If you learn nothing else from my book, I want you to learn that being in control is the most important part of this entire program. *You have to stop allowing other people and food to influence your health and wellness decisions.* Your friends and family may have a hard time with what you are doing. One reason is because they kind of envy your resolve. Deep down inside they wish they could do what you are doing, so they want you to fail, subconsciously, so they feel better about their failures. It's not really an intentional thing. It's a human thing. We generally have trouble feeling good about someone else's successes.

I was very lucky in that department. I had friends and family that totally supported me from the beginning all the way through. They watched me take charge of my life and change my behaviors. They encouraged me every step of the way. They continue to encourage me even after reaching my goal. They see that this is a true lifestyle change for me and they support me 100%. They are truly happy for my success. That's a great motivator, so the next step for you is:

Surround yourself with positive reinforcements!

Find people that can encourage you as you begin this program. Find friends and relatives that can be positive motivators, particularly at those weak times when you don't need someone to say: "Oh, one little piece isn't going to hurt you." You need someone to say, "You know you don't want it or need it. Look how well you have done so far." How they respond will determine the decisions you make about what you eat and if you stay on track or not. I have found that if you bring friends and family into the picture, you make yourself accountable to others for your success and/or failures. Sometimes, that is a motivator in itself. Sometimes, that accountability is all you need to keep you on track. We don't want to disappoint our friends and family. Or, we just don't want to have to tell them we blew it AGAIN!

You want their influence to help your efforts—not hurt your efforts. Remember, no matter what decisions you make, you are the one making them. And you are the one that either benefits or gets hurt by them. The final decisions are yours and the only person those decisions affect are you.

So:

Take charge.

Be in control.

Stay on track.

I just saw a commercial on television about yet another famous person who needed to lose weight, found a program that worked for her and is now promoting the weight loss program. That's great! I'm really happy for her. I'm sure that she has had the same struggles the rest of us have had. Just because she's rich and famous doesn't exclude her or anyone from the problem of being overweight. All I'm trying to say here is that they make it sound like now that THEY have tried the program and now that THEY have had success, we now can do it! It wasn't a good program or a successful program until they promoted it. Well, I'm here to tell you that one program does not fit all. Every person, every body, and physical system of every individual is just that—individual. We are all different from the inside out. The same foods, exercise, habits, training, whatever you put into your program needs to be tailored to YOU! Just because your next-door neighbor lost 50 pounds on a particular program, doesn't mean you'll lose 50 pounds. It doesn't even mean you'll lose any. I know there are tons of different programs out there and it all gets pretty overwhelming. I admit that I tried a few of them once or twice myself. But what I learned was this:

1. Diets don't work. At least not permanently. Because when you stop dieting, which you most definitely will do at some point, you will gain it all back and probably more.
2. All programs have similarities. They may vary slightly concerning what you eat, how much you eat, when you eat, if you have to take pills or supplements of some kind, etc, but they all tend to focus on 2 things: *food consumption* and *exercise*. Let's face it; any program will work if you eat the right foods and exercise. That's just a given.

I made a decision this time that as soon as I started losing the weight and had to replace my fat clothes with smaller sizes, I would get rid of them. I was never going back to that size—ever again! When I started, at 5' 1" tall, I was wearing 14's and 16's. Those were not my fat clothes—they were my only clothes. Now, believe it or not, my fat clothes would be a size 10, although I don't have a single size 10 anything in my closet. And even though a size 10 isn't a bad place to be, I don't plan on fitting back into them either! I've made it down to a size 4, believe it or not. Infact, I've never worn a size 4 in my entire life until now. How amazing is that?

All I'm saying is change your mind *AND* your habits. Don't even allow yourself the idea that you can always fall back on those "fat" clothes. Get them out of your mind—and out of your closet. You can do it. I have faith in you!

So, the time was fast approaching when I would have to stop losing the weight and start focusing on maintaining the weight loss. I had decided in my mind that I was never going back. All the fat clothes were gone. I finally got rid of them. Every time I lost weight before, the fat clothes stayed in the closet—just in case! It was always so easy to put a larger size on if the regular stuff was fitting a little too tight. My larger sizes were comfortable. They didn't make me feel so big. They felt "comfortable". And before I knew it, those were the clothes I was wearing every day—again. The pounds had come back and I was back where I had started. How depressing. Well, this time was definitely going to be different. The fat clothes would no longer be there for comfort. They would no longer be there to fall back on. They were gone for good.

To start over at my age would probably be futile. Where I was now was certainly going to be easier than starting again. So, I'm 40 pounds lighter. That's where I intend to stay for the rest of my life. What I've been doing up till now has been a total lifestyle change, so nothing needs to be different going forward. Actually, I did need to make one change and that was—are you ready for this?—I would actually have to start eating a little more or exercise a little less in order to maintain. Do you believe that? Honest! And then if a pound or two would creep on, I would catch it immediately and get it back off before 1 pound turned into 2, 2 pounds turned into 3, 3 pounds turned into 4 . . . . you see where I'm going with this. They call it LAPSE, RELAPSE, COLLAPSE. You want to catch it at the lapse, and never let it get to relapse!

*   *   *

Before I go any further, I think that we need to spend some serious time talking about exercise. I know I've already mentioned it several times and I know I've already told you the importance of exercise. What you need to understand before you get any further into this process is that without continuous exercise: before, during and after the desired weight loss, you will not be successful. Do you understand what I'm saying here? Even if you have lost the weight that you wanted, one way or another. Even if you have reached that desired goal. You will not have been successful or become successful or stay successful unless you have incorporated a regular exercise regiment along with everything else you are doing. I'm grateful that I learned this early on. I saw what happened when regular exercise was included with my program AND what happened when it was not included. You can eat the right stuff and lose the pounds, but if exercise is not part of all that you are doing, you may as well forget it. What I mean is that it has got to be as much a part of who you are as what you are (and are not) eating.

We are what we repeatedly do.
Excellence, therefore,
Is not an act but a habit.

Aristotle

I have to admit that I'm a pretty lucky lady because I just happen to LOVE exercise! Exercise is definitely a total part of my life, day in and day out. In fact, if I don't exercise one day, I truly feel like I've forgotten to do something major—like brush my teeth or something. I just feel weird. No matter how small or how short the time, I need to do some type of exercise to complete my day. Now, don't get me wrong, I have days just like everyone else when I absolutely do not feel like doing anything that resembles exercise. I can make up all kinds of great excuses for not exercising. But, when it's all said and done, if I choose not to exercise, I will and do regret that decision—every single time! I know that once I get started, I feel better almost immediately. And when I'm done, I am so much happier that I did it then if I didn't do it. That never changes. The hard part is getting motivated and staying motivated, and that's something we will talk about in more depth a little later on.

All I want you to understand now is that exercising on a regular basis is huge in the whole scheme of things where weight loss and weight management are concerned. So, for those times when you just don't feel like it—just do it !

I was talking to a girlfriend of mine the other day and as we were discussing dieting and weight loss and all that stuff, we started talking about the little changes that we decide to make when we finally psyched ourselves up to start losing weight. You try to think about what you can and can't live without when you start your program. You think about those morning lattes or those late night bags of popcorn, loaded with butter. Can you do without them? Can you cut back on them? What are you willing to give up or cut out temporarily until you get the pounds off? Let me tell you right now, that type of thinking will get you absolutely nowhere! I'm sorry to be the bearer of bad tidings, but you have to understand, this is not about temporary fixes or temporary changes. This is a total and complete lifestyle change. Have I said that before? Well, it bears repeating again, and again, and again and again, until it totally sinks in to that pretty little brain of yours. Whatever you decide to do now has to be for the rest of your life. I know that sounds too big to wrap your head around right now, but trust me, you will understand once you get started. You see, no matter what changes take place now, if you don't maintain those changes from here on out, your body will eventually go back to what it was use to before you started losing and the pounds will creep back on, one after the other, until one day you notice that you are not only back to where you started, but you may even be further behind all together. You don't want that to happen, do you?

Become one with your body! I know that sounds kind of Zen and I'm not into Zen, but the concept is this: Know your body inside and out by what you eat, what you drink, how you exercise and how your body responds to all of it. Let me see if I can explain this another way. Your body, up to this point, knows exactly what you are going to do day after day and it responds accordingly. Your body knows how much water it needs to retain because you either drink enough or too little. Your body knows how much fat to hold on to because of the food you consume day after day after day. So, by the same token, your body will respond to any changes you make. However, this is the trick. If you make drastic changes in what you eat or drink or how you exercise, your body will not make drastic changes at the same time. Your body is smarter than that. What it will do, is wait to see if this is just another one of those fly by night quick fixes that you've tried in the past, or if you are really serious about changing how you take care of yourself. It will take your body at least a couple of weeks before it will start to respond to the changes you are making. That means two things:

1. The changes need to be gradual.

2. The changes need to be consistent.

Your body needs to learn that the changes you are making now are not just temporary. Your body needs to know that this is a complete lifestyle change and once your body sees that this is the way it's going to be from here on out, then the necessary changes will start to take place. It won't take long. You will be amazed how well your body will respond to those changes once it is sure that those changes are for real. It will be at that point when you begin to work together with your body, taking in the right foods at the right time, in the right portions, drinking enough water, exercising. You will begin to function like a well oiled machine. Not to mention how awesome you will start to feel. I'm not kidding. Trust me on this!

Moving on . . . .

CHAPTER 4

Staying Motivated

We can do anything we want to do
if we stick to it long enough.

HELEN KELLER

I have talked to a lot of ladies since I started this program last July and they all seem to sing the same song: "I just can't seem to stay motivated". Each one seems to have a different reason, but the end result is the same—motivation. You start writing down what you eat every day and then one day you think, I can do this without writing it down. Or maybe you're out somewhere and you forget to take your food records with you or whatever you use to record your daily intake, and you think you can write it down when you get home. But, by the time you get home, you've pretty much forgotten what you ate and you find it hard to remember or even guess what you consumed. So, you think "I'll pick it back up tomorrow". Then tomorrow rolls around and something else happens that makes it difficult to record what you ate. Before you know it, a week has gone by, you've probably eaten way more than you should have and definitely way more than you would have if you had written it down every day. Are you getting the picture? This is how it starts and this is definitely how it will end.

Staying motivated is a job all in itself, but it is doable. My suggestion here is one simple word . . . .

VARIETY !!!

I know you've heard the saying "Variety is the spice of life". Well, where weight loss and exercise are concerned, this is definitely true. I know me and I know that I can get bored real easy if I'm doing the same thing over and over again. And that applies to just about anything in my life, not just weight loss. So I know that it's important for me to have a plethora of things to choose from when it's time for me to eat and exercise. Particularly when it comes to exercise.

First you need to find the types of exercise that you like. For me, it's bicycling, walking and step aerobics. That's a big enough selection to keep me interested and I have several variations for each that add to the variety. When my brother and I go bicycling, we change up our routes. The scenery changes, the distance changes. We may pick the same route, but do it in the opposite direction. That changes the whole perspective to me. When I walk, I can do the same thing. I can walk faster, walk slower, maybe even do a light jog. I can walk outside or inside on a treadmill. Lately, because I have so much more energy, I find that I can even actually run! That's amazing because I've never been able to run before. Step aerobics is my cold weather exercise because that I can do inside and at home. I enjoy it so much, I can throw it into my routine just about anytime, even if the weather is good outside. I have about 5 different videos and they are all different and work various parts of my body. One video is a basic step routine. Another one is a hip hop. Another is a power workout when I'm feeling really strong. Another is a floor exercise without the step. And the other one is circuit-training which incorporates stepping as well as weights. That one is a favorite because I get to add weights to my training. Weights are great because they not only add definition to your body, but weight training actually burns more calories. Did you know that?

Once you are far enough along in your exercise regiment, I highly suggest you add weights to your program. They don't have to be heavy. There just needs to be enough resistance to get your heart working a little harder. You can always increase the weight or the reps as you find yourself getting stronger.

* *

Desire is the starting point of all achievement,

not

a hope, not a wish, but a keen

pulsating desire which transcends everything.

Napoleon Hill

* *

Now, I just want to stop here for one minute and acknowledge someone in my life that has helped me to stay motivated. Actually, I have two people. The first person is my brother. He has been an amazing support for me throughout this whole program. He was the first one to notice the changes in my face. I've been extremely lucky because my brother has been in athletics his whole life, so he knows a lot about weight training and what is and isn't important. He has encouraged me every step of the way. And whenever we're out somewhere together, he is my biggest cheerleader! You have no idea how great that makes me feel.

The second person is a coworker of mine. She has been amazing with her encouragement and interest in what I've accomplished. Every week, at the beginning of my program, the first thing she would do is ask how much weight I had lost. I was always so excited to tell her another pound came off, and then another, and then another. Just knowing she was going to ask every week kept me motivated to keep losing. Even now she continues to tell me how proud she is of what I have accomplished.

What that tells me is we need people to be accountable to for what we are doing and not doing. Believe me, you don't want to have to tell that person that you blew it again and again, or that you gained another pound instead of losing it. You want to be able to tell them how great you're doing. That's motivation!

As I mentioned at the beginning of this chapter, you need to add variety to the food you eat as well as your exercise. There are so many wonderful things out there that you can eat, and you need to find those foods that you like best. Nobody wants to chew on a raw carrot stick if they hate carrots. Know what I mean? If you love raw carrots, then that's a no brainer. Find the foods you like, choose the right portion per serving and incorporate it into your diet.

I'm a little different than most people. If truth be told, my diet is pretty basic, but for me, it works. Every week I choose a meat, a vegetable and a fruit. Sometimes I choose two vegetables and two fruits. Then I cook one day a week and eat the same thing for that entire week. I usually cook on Sunday and spend several hours preparing the food and then placing it into single serving containers. Then, every morning, I grab a meat, a vegetable and a fruit and that's my main meal for the afternoon. I also have something for breakfast and I also add a couple of single serving snacks for in between. Remember, I told you that once you have set your body on a regular routine of eating right and exercising, you will need to eat more often. I usually have something to eat every couple of hours. It seems like I'm eating all the time now, but because my body is burning more and because my metabolism has been sped up, I need to continue to consume more food to keep my body going. If your body is not taking in enough nourishment, you will be hungry and when you're hungry, it's easy to eat the wrong things or too much.

There's one more trick I learned that I want to share with you as well. I found out that when you feel hungry, it's possible your body really just needs water. Did you know that? Well, try this: The first time you think you're hungry, drink an 8 ounce glass of water. Then wait for 30 minutes. If you still feel hungry, then eat something. I guarantee that some of those times, the water will do the trick and eating will not be necessary. Think of the number of times you have put something in your mouth simply because you thought you were hungry. We just took care of that problem, didn't we?

LET'S REGROUP FOR A MINUTE . . . .

If all of this seems a bit overwhelming and you just don't know where to start, let me offer a bit of constructive advice:

1. Start small.
2. Make small, attainable goals first.
3. As goals are reached, keep adding more goals
4. Goals that are reached are very powerful and can give you the added strength and encouragement you need to keep moving forward with your progress.
5. Make your goals permanent, not temporary.
6. Whatever goals you choose to start, start them with the intention that they are now part of your lifestyle. Positive changes do not work if they are not done consistently and permanently.
7. Remember, it takes approximately 21 days for something to become a habit. Think about those small goals in terms of making them habits. Once they become part of your daily and/or weekly routine, they become easier to continue. At that point, you'll be surprised how much you will need them in your routine.
8. Give yourself a break.
9. Stop beating up on yourself when you slip. Remember: Lapse, Relapse, Collapse! Catch it at Lapse and don't let it go any further. Pick yourself up, brush yourself off and start all over again!
10. YOU CAN DO THIS !
11. If it's important to you, you'll find a way. If it's not, you'll find an excuse!
12. YOU CAN DO THIS !

13. YOU CAN DO THIS !

And just in case you didn't get it the first *THREE* times,

YOU CAN DO THIS !!!

CHAPTER 5

Eating Sensibly

I was watching one of those commercials I had mentioned before and the person promoting the weight loss program said something like this: "I have been successful because I am taking this product along with sensible eating and exercise". I hate when they say that. Do you know **why** I hate when they say that? Because you don't need to take any product at all as long as you eat sensibly and exercise. **A***nybody* can lose weight if they eat sensibly and exercise.

Okay, there it is!

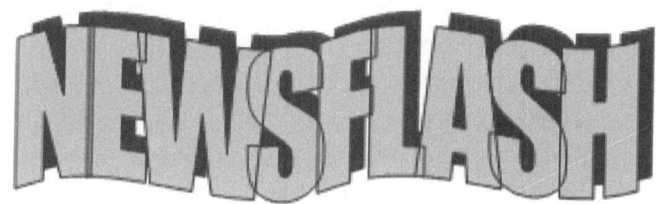

SENSIBLE EATING AND EXERCISE *WILL* PROMOTE WEIGHT LOSS AND GOOD HEALTH

That's the big secret that everybody has been keeping to themselves all this time. Listen to me, you don't need this diet pill or that diet pill or this diet drink or that diet drink. All you need is to eat sensibly and exercise regularly. That's your winning combo. And *It's guaranteed 100%.*

I don't think we've talked much about sensible eating yet, so let's dive into that part. Sensible eating includes portion control. In addition to eating the right stuff, you also have to make sure you're eating the right portion. Even good food can be bad if you eat too much of it. You have to learn the right foods to eat and how much of it to eat. I'm here to tell you that most people haven't got a clue what "portion control" is all about. That's the tricky part of weight loss and weight management. How much really is a serving? I've talked to a bunch of people and they are shocked when they find out that one meal figures out to be more like 3 or 4 meals when you look at the number of servings they are eating. And then they get all nervous and think there is no way they could cut those meals up into 3 or 4 smaller meals and be satisfied. Well, that's the beauty of this. Believe it or not, I actually eat more now than I ever did when I was heavier. I'm actually eating smaller servings (portion control) but I'm eating more often. With portion control and regular exercise, you will speed up your metabolism and burn more calories at a much faster pace. For me, that means I can eat more often as long as my portions are smaller so that my body burn the calories continuously. Remember, your body is paying very close attention to what you eat, how much you eat, and when you eat. Each of those attribute to how much fat your body will burn and how much fat your body will hold on to. The idea is that you are burning more than you are taking in. That's where the weight loss part comes in. Calories out vs. calories in. How many calories are you eating and how many are you burning? If your body is not burning the calories faster than the calories you are taking in, then weight loss will not happen.

As I've said before, it's vital that you understand exactly how your body works. All of these things work together to give you the best formula for your personal needs. Don't worry about what Susie next door is doing or how much weight Patty lost in just a month. You need to worry about YOU! What do you need to do to be successful. And success is not just measured in what's happening now . . . . real success is measured in how are you doing in 6 months, in a year, 5 years from now. All of this hard work is not a quick fix and it's not temporary. This is the rest of your life we're talking about, so what you accomplish now will sustain you throughout the remainder of your life. And the longer you do it, the easier it all becomes. All of these changes you are making now are gradually becoming habits for you, so as time goes on, you will do all of these things without even really thinking about it. They will become second nature to you.

And let's face it, isn't that what we all really want. We want this hard work to become less like hard work and more like every day living. Habits and routines are hard to break once they become habits and routines, so that's what you want. Instead of bad habits and bad routines, why wouldn't you want to replace those with good habits and good routines?

I use to envy this one lady I worked with who practiced portion control every day of her life. Whenever we had desserts or special treats at work, she would take a very small piece or bite and be totally satisfied. I, on the other hand, had to have a huge piece of whatever it was and totally pig out. Of course, after I ate it, the satisfaction was gone and I really regretted it. Have you ever felt that way? Why do we do that to ourselves, time and time again? But now it's different. I can either look at something like that and not have it at all, or I can take a very small piece and be totally happy with that very small piece. And you know what else? After I've had that very small piece, I'm really quite satisfied. There's no need for beating myself up for eating it because it wasn't significant. I don't need any more and the desire is gone. What a great feeling. The other great thing is that I can do that kind of thing more often because I'm not over indulging each time.

This is the habit I suggest you start making a part of your lifestyle as soon as possible . . . .

PORTION CONTROL

As you are learning to eat better foods, even if you find yourself still eating things you probably shouldn't, if they are in smaller portions, it will become easier to let those foods go and replace them with the good stuff!

To help you with portion control, let me suggest something I found to be extremely helpful. Measure your food and put it in single serving containers. There are a variety of storage containers out there that actually show the measurements on the side of each container. They come in a variety of sizes, but I prefer the 1 to 2 cup containers. For instance, when I measure out my cereal for the day, it goes in a 1-cup container. From the side panel of the box I know how many calories are in a 1 cup serving with 1 cup of milk. I do the same thing with my lunches. Everything I eat is placed in single serving containers. It makes it much easier to keep track of my calorie intake for each meal. It also makes portion control effortless. It takes the guesswork out of it. By the time I leave work to go home, I know how many calories I have taken in and how many calories I can consume that evening.

And that reminds me of another trick I found very useful. This was actually the first real change I made when I first started my program. I knew that a big part of my problem was eating at night before I went to bed. So, I decided that I would stop eating at 8:00 p.m. every night. Whatever I was going to consume for that day had to be consumed before 8:00 p.m. For many of us that's not an easy change to make, but I did it and I found it to be a big part of my success in losing weight. I never realized how many calories I was mindlessly consuming in the course of the evening. And a lot of it was just before going to bed. I wasn't even giving my body enough time to really digest what I had eaten. Too much food on my stomach also contributed to a very poor night's sleep.

Find the foods that you like best. Make them a regular part of your menu. Incorporate other foods in as well. Learn to eat things you may not have tried before. There are fruits and vegetables out there that you may never have thought about trying, but once you do, you'll be pleasantly surprised to find out you actually like them!

A very dear friend of mine back east always seemed to have a wonderful variety of fruit on her table. One day she told me I should try a mango. I thought to myself, "You have got to be kidding. What would I possibly do with a mango?" She told me to just try it and see. So, one day I bought a mango. I really didn't have any idea how to even cut it open. I looked it up in my Betty Crocker cookbook, peeled it and cut it up into pieces like it showed in the book. Then I took a taste. Wow! I was hooked. I am now just about addicted to mangoes. I can't seem to live without them. How great is it to be hooked on a mango? I feel the same way about a couple of other fruits and even a few vegetables.

I can remember when I was addicted to chocolate. In fact, I was a *chocoholic*! Honest. I was addicted in the worst way. And I couldn't just eat a little piece of chocolate. I had to eat it until it was practically coming out my ears. If I bought a bag of M&M's, I ate the whole bag. And it was usually a big bag! If I bought cookies or something like that, I couldn't stop at one or two. I had to eat it until it was gone. Portion control was foreign to me.

Once I incorporated good foods into my diet, I found that I really liked them. If you can fill your cupboards with good things to eat, even if you over indulge once in a while, you're still over indulging on something that's good for you. And, that's not all bad. I still love chocolate, but I eat it very sparing these days. And believe it or not, I don't miss it!

Look for those bad habits and eliminate them from your daily routine. Start setting up some new, better habits for eating the right kinds of foods. You have choices. You can either keep doing things the way you always have and nothing will change, or you can decide to do what's best for your future health.

The changes you will see and experience are amazing. In case you need a little incentive to get started, here are just a few:

1. You will sleep so much better
2. You will have more energy during the day
3. Food simply tastes better
4. You will experience better digestion
5. Drinking more water will give you clearer skin
6. You'll definitely need to shop for new clothes—smaller sizes!

Need I say more?

PERSEVERANCE IS NOT A LONG RACE;

IT IS MANY SHORT RACES

ONE AFTER ANOTHER

WALTER ELLIOTT

Let's continue . . . .

CHAPTER 6

Exercise 101

If you will remember, further back in the book, I told you that without exercise, you may as well not start this program at all. Well, I'm saying it again. Without putting a full-time exercise program into your daily routine, you might as well not even bother losing weight! This is serious ladies: because exercise is really the secret weapon of this entire regiment. One way or another, everyone can lose weight. Eventually, you'll find something that works for you and the pounds will come off. But here's the thing: the inches won't and that's the difference between simply losing weight and changing your entire body.

I truly did not believe I could change the way my body was shaped. At my age, I thought it was impossible. I had developed that extra weight around the middle and I hated the way all of my clothes fit and looked. I was a larger woman on the top so I had to buy larger sizes just so they wouldn't cling to me. I hated the way that looked. There's nothing worse than seeing a woman with that extra weight around the middle with a top that's too tight. You can see every roll from top to bottom. It's so unattractive. Larger tops hide the rolls, but they certainly don't look attractive, and they don't make you feel attractive either.

I want to share something with you about myself that I think will help you to understand where I'm coming from. I want you to picture what I am saying so that you will understand that I know what I'm talking about. For as long as I can remember, I have had extremely large breasts. They were a tremendous hindrance my entire life. I was only 5' 1" tall in stature, short waisted, with large breasts. Not a great combination for high self esteem. All the time I was growing up, I was always very self-conscious about my breasts because that's all that anyone ever saw of me. At least it seemed like it because it was the only place on my body they were looking at. I loved athletics, but because of the size of my breasts, I was extremely limited with what I could do. I certainly couldn't run. Back then, it was almost impossible to find a bra that fit properly, let alone could give you total support. Thank God that's not the case today.

Okay, so I had large breasts, I was short-waisted, and I had a pretty big belly on me. My mother was built pretty much the same way, so I figured it was just a part of my heredity. Over the years, I tried to stay in shape. I continued to stay active, exercising, playing whatever types of sports I could handle. If truth be told, I was pretty limited with the amount of weight I could lose because the smaller the rest of my body got, the larger my breasts got. You heard me correctly. I remember one other time in my life when I lost a fair amount of weight. My bra size was already 42DD. Well, believe it or not, I reduced my bra size around, but increased my cup size to a 40DDD. I was mortified! I didn't need them any bigger! What was I to do?

I continued to try and take care of myself, trying to eat right and exercise, but my breasts were really becoming a problem. The last straw was when I started taking Pilates at a local health club where I lived back east. I loved Pilates and was having a great time strengthening my core and my legs, but I reached what seemed to be a plateau. I couldn't do more or get any better at it because my breasts were getting in the way. That was when I decided I would have a breast reduction. I tell you all of this for you to understand the new challenge set before me once I had the breast reduction. Let me just say it was the best thing I could have done for myself, but that's a whole different story we can tackle in another book. This book is talking about what my midsection looked like after my reduction. My breasts had been so large for so long, I never knew exactly what the rest of my body looked like under my breasts.

After I healed from my surgery, I had all this extra fat that just stuck out around my middle. At that moment, I wasn't quite sure which was worse. At least with large breasts, you can harness them. My middle was just sticking out there for everyone to see. I felt I could wear smaller tops because of my breast reduction, but still found I looked awful because of my large midsection. And after I thought about it, I realized the only way I was going to fix that part of my body was with exercise. I knew it wasn't going to be easy, but I knew it was necessary. Like I said before, I never really thought it was all going to go away, but if I could at least reduce it or tighten it a little, anything would be a plus for me. I told you all of that to say this: exercise is paramount in your weight loss and weight management program. I never realized just how successful I could be with reducing that midsection with regular exercise, along with a good eating program.

You see, this is the thing: when you diet to lose weight, if you don't incorporate exercise along with the change in eating habits, your body will pull from the muscle, not the fat. That's not good. Your goal is to build muscle and reduce fat. If you add regular exercise, your body will respond to the routine by eliminating the fat that has collected and muscle will replace it. Let me just mention right here that that's also the reason why when you step on the scales you might see that you have put on weight instead of lost it. How discouraging is that? Well, don't be. Once you start getting the fat off and replacing it with muscle, the pounds will begin to fall off. And it's at that point when you start to see the total reshaping of your body. It's amazing when that happens.

I still have a bit around the middle to get off, but I'm working at it. I've said this before but it bears repeating: a woman's midsection is not an easy area to reduce. It will take regular, targeted exercises. My body is now much more proportioned from top to bottom. My top half fits with my bottom half. My bra is now a 36 instead of a 42 and I've taken about 8 inches off of my waist. Those tops that use to cling to my body are now literally hanging on me. I had to buy new tops, only this time I don't mind them clinging to me because I truly like what I see.

This is what I think about EXERCISE:

E XPERIENCE

X CELLENCE

E VERY DAY

R EGARDLESS OF THE

C HALLENGES THAT

I NTERFERE WITH THE

S UCCESS OF YOUR

E FFORTS

EXPERIENCE EXCELLENCE EVERY DAY REGARDLESS OF THE CHALLENGES THAT INTERFERE WITH THE SUCCESS OF YOUR EFFORTS.

And believe me, there will be challenges every single day that interfere with the success of your efforts. Count on it! Just when you think you've made it through one obstacle, there will be another one waiting just around the corner. How you approach and handle those obstacles and challenges will make all the difference in how successful you will be. But the results you will see and feel are so worth it. My hope is that you will find an exercise routine that not only works for you, but one that you find fun and motivating. Isn't that what we've been talking about throughout this book? This entire weight loss and weight management program has to be tailored to fit you and your body. It needs to be a program you can start with and stay with. It needs to be a program with variety so that you can stay motivated and enjoy what you are doing. This program needs to be a program that will stay with you for the rest of your life.

And, feel free to change and modify the program at any time. If something you are doing isn't working for you, don't keep doing it. Change it. Remove something from your exercise routine if you don't feel motivated or find that you dread doing it. I am always looking to vary my exercise program because I get bored really easy. So I have to change it up. If you read about a new exercise that targets a certain part of the body that you haven't been focusing on, by all means, give it a try. If you like it, incorporate it into your program. If not, don't worry, there are plenty of other exercises you can try until you find the ones that work for you. When the program you choose becomes a personal one, that's when you will find that it's easy to stay with it.

Perseverance allows you to get back on track when you hit a detour.

—Catherine Pulsifer

Perseverance, Excellence, Success, Desire. These are words that will determine if you make it or you don't. How bad do you want it? How important is it to you? Will your life be okay without it? I challenge you to make a life for yourself that is forever changed. One accomplishment will set your life on a path of continuous success. Time after time you will set your goals and reach them.

CHAPTER 7

Good Dessert Substitutes

This is probably my most favorite subject: **DESSERT !!!**

I so love dessert, sweets, particularly chocolate. However, I do have to mention that since I changed my eating habits, I am happy to report that my taste for sweets has changed as well. I'm not saying I don't crave sweets—I still do. The difference now is that I know how to put those cravings into check and not give in to them every time they rear their ugly head. The difference now is that I know that I can enjoy my sweets on special occasions and when I do, I truly enjoy them so much more because it's not an every day thing. Those rare times when I treat myself to something I wouldn't normally eat, I will choose something that is truly decadent, rich and oh, so special. That's why they call it a treat.

This is very important for you to understand. I'm not telling you never to eat certain things. What I'm telling you is "everything in moderation". If you find yourself buying that caramel chocolate latte with double whip cream every morning, maybe you should think about just having that once a week—or better yet—once a month!

My problem was and still is every time I finish eating, my body wants something sweet. Growing up, my mother was an amazing cook. Everything she made, she made from scratch. And every day, after every meal, there was always some kind of dessert. We had cake, pies, cookies, you name it. After lunch, there was usually a tin filled with chocolate chip cookies or a pan of brownies. After dinner, there was normally a double layer cake or chocolate cream pie with homemade whipped topping. I didn't have to think twice about it. It was normal for me to eat my meal and finish it off with whatever wonderful dessert she had made that day. My body got use to it. My body looked forward to it and that was a routine I maintained most of my life. Of course, I've also struggled with my weight most of my life and now I understand why. I can honestly tell you that no matter how much I ate, no matter how full I was, I probably couldn't put another bite of food in my mouth, I was so full I could hardly move, but trust me when I tell you *I always had room for dessert!*

Now, your problem may not be sweets. You may crave salty things like chips. Or maybe breads are your downfall. Whatever it is, we're all in the same boat. We need to learn to control those cravings and to help us with that, we need to find good and healthy replacements. There are a lot of good foods on the market today. I am so grateful for that. I also found I actually changed my cravings to accommodate those good and healthy substitutes. It doesn't mean I don't still want those decadent desserts. What it does mean is that I can be totally satisfied with the substitutes I have chosen and that is huge for me. Let me see if I can give you a couple of examples:

One of the first things I can think of is ice cream. I am happy to report that over the years, I actually found that I prefer frozen yogurt instead of real ice cream. For someone who loves ice cream as much as I do, that was a big deal in itself. But I could actually sit and eat entire half gallon of frozen yogurt in one sitting. No, really! I'm not kidding! Portion control was a really big deal with this one, but Skinny Cows have saved me. I love Skinny Cows. The ice cream sandwiches are my favorite because they automatically help me with portion control. I have learned to enjoy eating just one Skinny Cow ice cream sandwich. Why? Because I know that I can have another one tomorrow, and the next day and the next day. I don't have to deprive myself of something I like. I just have to learn to control how much of it I eat.

There are really a lot of good frozen dessert type treats at your local grocery store. Let me suggest that you try a few. If you love ice cream type products like I do, try some of the frozen yogurts or sorbets. I really love sorbets, too, but they usually come in pint containers. Now, I know that a pint is no where near as much as a half gallon, but for me to sit and eat an entire pint would not be difficult, but one pint normally contains about 4 servings, so that's not good portion control. Because my cravings were so severe, I've had to be extremely severe with my adjustments. You may not be as bad as me, so adjust according to your own requirements. Sadly, I learned that even a pint is difficult for me to resist, so if it doesn't come in single serving containers, I can't buy it. It's as simple as that. Now Weight Watchers has come out with single serving ice cream desserts that I truly enjoy. One little container has proven to satisfy my cravings and once again, I can enjoy a single serving every day if I wish. I was never much of a fruity type dessert kind of girl, but fruit has definitely become a big part of my life, so fruit in desserts is a better option for me now. My brother turned me on to a strawberry frozen fruit bar that is out of this world. It has huge chunks of strawberries running all through the bar. They are so good and only 80 calories a bar! Once in a while, I even eat two of them! If strawberries aren't your thing, there are all kinds of fruity fruit bars in your grocer's freezer: orange, grape, lime, there's even a coconut one I really love! I'm sure there is one that you will find truly satisfying.

I really could go on and on with my dessert choices. This has probably been the biggest obstacle for me with this entire weight loss and weight management program. But I am so happy to report that your eating habits and eating choices can change just like your regular eating habits can. It's what you get your body and taste buds to get use to that make the difference between success and failure. You can make better choices and be satisfied without feeling like you're depriving yourself of something.

I don't crave sweets like I use to. My body craves the good substitutes. My body now responds accordingly to the types of foods I give it. When I eat something I'm not use to eating, my body lets me know. Sometimes I feel more lethargic. Sometimes

I simply feel sick to my stomach. My system just isn't use to eating some of those things I use to eat on a regular basis. My body now wants more fruits, more vegetables, more good things because that's what it is use to NOW! Remember I told you that this program will cause you to become more aware of what your body needs and doesn't need. Pay attention to what your body is telling you. That's how you know whether what you are doing is helping or hurting your progress. Bad habits are so hard to break and good habits take at least 21 days to become habits, so get started. Your success depends upon the choices you make for now and years to come.

SUCCESS IS THE SUM OF SMALL EFFORTS, REPEATED DAY IN AND DAY OUT.

ROBERT COLLIER

CHAPTER 8

Useful Websites

Most of us are computer savvy, so we know that there are websites out there for just about anything you could possibly want or need. I have searched an abundance of websites looking for information that I can use to help me with exercise choices as well as food choices. As I have said time and time again throughout this book, you have to find what works best for you. I can only offer those websites and information that I have acquired over this last year that I think have been useful for me. But with the information I am giving you, you can dig even deeper or search even further and probably find a lot more. And more importantly, find information that will work best for you. Whatever information you locate, whatever websites you chose, use the information that works for you and discard what doesn't. There's a lot of stuff out there and it all can get a bit overwhelming, but as you progress with your program, you will learn what truly works for you and what doesn't.

Here are just a few websites I think may be useful:

www.calorieking.com

I found this website to be most helpful to me. I kept it as a quick reference on my computer so that I could always look up and see almost exactly how many calories I am eating of something. This is an extensive database of every kind of food you can think of with several portion sizes so you can get an accurate count of calories going in. This website offers a lot more, but just counting my calories and helping with portion control was huge for me.

www.fitday.com

This website is very similar to calorie king and offers pretty much the same information. You can join either one of these free of charge or pay if you want more involvement. You can keep a daily journal, which has also proven to be a very effective way to keep yourself accountable. It also gives you the opportunity to track how well you are doing on a regular basis. Both of these websites allow you to use a little or a lot of information. Whatever is most helpful for your progress.

www.sparkpeople.com

This website is a community of people that are dealing with the same weight loss problems as you. You can talk to people who may be struggling with the same things you are and gives you a chance to make connections with them to share your thoughts and ideas if you so choose. This website also offers a ton of information for whatever you may need or want. There are a couple things I like about this website: one is that they send regular emails about all kinds of things. The email caption allows me to see if it's information I want or don't want. I can read it or not. It's up to me, but the information comes to you on a regular basis, so if you don't like receiving a lot of emails, you might not want to utilize that part of this one. The other thing I like about this website is it gives you regular exercise information. And the best part is they show a demonstration of how to actually perform the exercise. If you are targeting a particular part of your body that needs work, and you don't know what exercise would be best, this website probably has it and can show you how to do it. There's also a section with videos that you can actually follow the exercises whenever you want.

www.calorie-count.com

This is still another website similar to Calorieking and Fitday. It's worth it to look at all of these types of websites to see which one is the best fit for you. One may give you more of what you are looking for, or any one of them may be equally as useful. You decide.

www.lowsodiumcooking.com

This is a website that offers a lot of good information about sodium, the good and the bad of it, and offers low sodium recipes if you're interested.

If you're anything like me, I have had to battle with high blood pressure and because of that, I've had to be very careful with my salt intake. Let me just say right here and now, I believe everyone should be careful with their salt (sodium) intake. There is a ton of sodium in packaged and processed foods, so I always recommend that you prepare your own meals. Buying already prepared foods may be quick and easy, but it certainly isn't healthy. When you're reading the labels in the grocery store, and you see the calorie count and the fat grams, make sure you take a look at the sodium count as well. You will be amazed—and shocked—to see just how high it is per serving! Be very, very careful with your purchases. It may not be a big problem right now in your life, but I guarantee it will be later on if you aren't careful now.

www.lowsaltcooking.com

This is another website pretty much like the low sodium one I just mentioned.

www.beinglive.com

If you have trouble losing weight on your own and need a little help, this website offers a personal success coaching program. I believe the program has a membership cost, but you may find that what they can offer you is worth the fee. Check it out.

www.prevention.com

This website is a duplicate of the hard copy issue you can buy in the grocery store. I happen to love Prevention magazine. It is always jam packed with valuable as well as interesting information about health and wellness. If you don't want the hard copies sitting around and taking up space, you may find the website is a better choice. That way you can pick and choose what you want to read, when you want to read it.

www.about.com

This is one of those websites where you simply type in what you are looking for, and they will direct you to another website to help you find your answer. They advertise 750 experts ready and willing to help you with whatever you might need. Could prove to be a valuable option if you are having trouble finding an answer to something really specific.

www.nutritiondata.com

Still another nutrition, food, calorie, etc., type website that can offer tons of information. I'm sure there are still many more I haven't even found, but maybe in your searches you will find one I haven't mentioned that works even better for you. Let me know what you come up with. I'd be interested to hear.

www.nal.usda.gov/fnic/foodcomp/search

If you are a true intellectual, you might find this website interesting. This is the National Nutrient Database. Need I say more?

www.nwcr.ws/default.htm

This is the National Weight Control Registry. To be perfectly honest I have not spent any time on this website as yet, but now that I have reached my goal weight, I think I'm ready to register here. This is an ongoing study of people who have lost a certain amount of weight and have maintained that weight loss for a period of time. You might want to participate in the study if you meet their qualifications.

www.wisegeek.com

This website's name kind of speaks for itself. This one simply allows you to ask common questions and get common answers. I haven't really tried this one because there seems to be a lot of other websites that have answered most all of my questions already. But, you never know, you may find it helpful along the way.

Like I said before, there are a ton more websites I haven't even mentioned or looked into. I'm sure you will find others all on your own. The point is that you're not alone in this endeavor. There is so much helpful information out there. Please avail yourself to what the Internet has to offer. Remember, you can always contact me if you have a questions or just need someone to talk to.

I have also added a page on Portion Control to help you with making the right portion selections. There's a page that lists Super Foods. These are items you definitely want to include in your diet on a regular basis. You don't have to eat all of them, but try as many as you can. You'll be surprised how good they are—and how good they are for you. Lastly, I made a page for your food and exercise journal. Copy this page and use it on a daily basis.

Well, I think that's just about all I have to say on the subject of weight loss and weight management. This isn't a huge book so mark it up, highlight the things you want to remember or the sections that you need to refer back to from time to time. Read the book over and over and over again until you have made these changes a habit. This is the rest of your life. This is your future. It's starting to look a lot brighter, isn't it?

Good Luck.

God Bless.

VEGETABLES	FRUITS	PROTEINS
Asparagus	Apples	Almonds
Avocados	Apricots	Beef, lean
Beets	Bananas	Black beans
Bell peppers	Black olives	Cashews
Broccoli	Blackberries	Chicken, skinless
Brussels sprouts	Blueberries	Chickpeas
Cabbage	Cantaloupe	Egg whites
Carrots	Cherries	Eggs
Cauliflower	Cranberries	Fish, unbreaded
Collard greens	Figs	Flaxseed
Crimini mushrooms	Grapefruit	Garbanzo beans
Cucumbers	Grapes	Hemp seeds
Eggplant	Honeydew melon	Hummus
Garlic	Kiwifruit	Kidney beans
Green beans	Lemons	Lima beans
Kale	Limes	Lentils
Mustard greens	Nectarines	Miso
Onions	Oranges	Navy beans
Peas	Papaya	Nuts
Portobello	Peaches	Peanut butter, natural
mushrooms	Pears	Peanuts
Potatoes	Pineapple	Pinto beans
Rainbow chard	Plums	Pork, lean
Romaine lettuce	Prunes	Pumpkin seeds
Shiitake mushrooms	Raisins	Salmon, canned or
Spinach	Raspberries	fresh
Summer squash	Strawberries	Seafood, unbreaded
Sweet potatoes	Watermelon	Sesame seeds
Swiss chard		Soybeans
Tomatoes		Sunflower seeds
Turnip greens		Tahini
Winter squash		Tempeh
Yams		Tofu
		Tuna, canned or
		fresh
		Turkey, skinless

CALCIUM-RICH FOODS

Almond milk
Cheese, low fat
Cottage cheese, low fat
Milk, skim or 1%
Orange juice with calcium
Rice milk
Soy milk
Yogurt with active cultures, low fat

GRAINS

Amaranth
Arborio rice
Barley
Brown rice
Buckwheat
Bulgur
Corn
Jasmine
Millet
Oats
Quinoa
Rye
Spelt
Triticale
Wheat berries
Whole grain breads, cereal, pasta
Whole wheat breads, cereal, pasta
Wild Rice

Veggie burgers
Walnuts
Wild game, skinless

MISCELLANEOUS

Canola oil
Dark chocolate
Green tea
Olive oil

PORTION CONTROL REFERENCE GUIDE

GRAINS: Aim for 6-11 servings each day. Choose whole grains whenever possible.

EXAMPLES	ONE SERVING EQUALS	COMPARE TO
Bread	1 ounce (1 small slice, 1/2 bagel, 1/2 bun)	Index card
Cooked Grains	1/2 cup cooked oats, rice, pasta	Billiard ball
Dry cereal	1/2 cup flakes, puffed rice, shredded wheat	Billiard ball

FRUITS & VEGETABLES: Aim for 5-9 total servings each day. Choose fresh fruits and veggies whenever possible.

EXAMPLES	ONE SERVING EQUALS	COMPARE TO
Raw fruit	1/2 cup raw, canned, frozen fruit	Billiard ball
Dried fruit	1/4 cup raisins, prunes, apricots	An egg
Juice	6 oz 100% fruit or vegetable juice	Hockey puck
Raw vegetables	1 cup leafy greens, baby carrots	Baseball
Cooked vegetables	1/2 cup cooked broccoli, potatoes	Billiard ball

MEAT & BEANS: Aim for 2-3 servings each day. Choose lean meats and plant proteins whenever possible.

EXAMPLES	ONE SERVING EUALS	COMPARE TO
Meat & Tofu	2-3 oz cooked beef, poultry, fish, tofu	Deck of cards
Beans	1/2 cup cooked beans, split peas, legumes	Billiard ball
Nuts & Seeds	2 Tbsp nuts, seeds, or nut butters	Ping pong ball

DAIRY: Aim for 2-3 servings of calcium-rich foods each day. Choose low- or non-fat products whenever possible.

EXAMPLES	ONE SERVING EQUALS	COMPARE TO
Cheese	1 ounce or 1 thin slice of cheese	A pair of dice
Milk	1 cup milk, yogurt, soy milk	Baseball

FATS & OILS: Eat fats and oils sparingly and in small portions. Choose heart-healthy fats whenever possible.

EXAMPLES	ONE SERVING EQUALS	COMPARE TO
Fat & Oil	1 tsp butter, margarine, oil	One die

FOOD & EXERCISE JOURNAL

DAY	_____	DATE	____ / ____ / ____
AMOUNT	FOOD & BEVERAGES	CALORIES	COMMENTS
TOTAL			

PHYSICAL ACTIVITY DIARY

DATE	DAY	MINUTES	TYPE OF ACIVITY

CLOSING NOTES

I was just reading an article about preparing for retirement. Now, I know that I am a little ways away from retirement. A little ways away in age that is, but a long ways away in financial stability. However, it is a time of my life I am certainly preparing for. And the great part about it for me now is that I know I am so much healthier and so much happier at this stage of my life than I was 20 or more years ago. I feel great, I look great (at least I think I do), and I'm ready to try new things.

Any age, whether you are young or old, is a great time to start taking better care of yourself. It doesn't matter what age you are, now is never too late to start better health care. The benefits are huge. Remember, set small, attainable goals and when you've reached them, set new ones. Make gradual changes that are easy to start and easy to stick with. And above all else, don't beat yourself up when you slip. Nobody is perfect, so give yourself a break. You are your own worst critic, and women have proven to be the hardest on themselves. Ladies, you are God's amazing creatures. There is no one like you! Don't you deserve the very best life has to offer? Don't you want to feel great and look great every day for the rest of your life? Well, today is the day. Start now and be amazed at all you can achieve.

* * * * * * * * * * * * * * * * * *

This is not the end of my journey. What I have started here will stay with me for the rest of my life. I feel like a million bucks and I'm ready to take on the world. Are you? Let's do this together. If I can help you in any way with your program, please feel free to contact me at: bljackson57@gmail.com. I would love to hear from you.

Thanks for listening.

ACKNOWLEDGEMENTS

First I want to thank my co-worker, Cherie Callero, who has been such an encouragement to me throughout my weight loss program. Cherie walked with me Monday through Thursday without fail. Every one step with her long legs equaled at least two of mine, so she continued to push me to do better. When the weather was iffy, Cherie still got out there with me. There were even times she would come in on her Fridays off just to walk with me. What a trooper! Thanks Cherie for being such a good friend.

Second I want to thank my brother, Jim Jackson, who has been my biggest cheerleader. He always took time out of his busy schedule to go bike riding with me so I could easily stay on track. He taught me things about my health and my body I never would have learned any other way. And he always bragged on me every time we were around friends and family. He always made me feel good about what I had done. My brother has also taught me over the years that there is nothing you can't do if you apply yourself. I am so honored to be his Baby Sister!

Lastly, and most important, I want to thank my Lord and Savior, Jesus Christ. Without His strength and unconditional love for me, I would not be the woman I am today. I am so thankful.

I prayed long and hard for God to give me strength and determination to stick with this weight loss program. And when my words matched my heart, God went to work. As He has always done in my life, He answered my prayers and gave me more than I would ever have expected.

His plans for my life have been amazing so far. I can't wait to see what lies ahead. The person I am today is definitely going to enjoy the rest of my life so much more!

YOU ONLY LIVE ONCE, BUT IF YOU LIVE RIGHT, ONCE IS ENOUGH.

Joe E. Lewis

www.ingramcontent.com/pod-product-compliance
Lightning Source LLC
Chambersburg PA
CBHW031328290526
45784CB00014B/2432